America and Abortion

Two Nations within One Country

Pedro M. Anderson

America and Abortion:

Two Nations within One Country

Pedro M. Anderson

Table of Contents

Copyright

DEDICATION

This work is dedicated to the Almighty God for helping me throughout writing this book and also this work is dedicated to anyone out there who is struggling with emotional and psychological challenges

BACKGROUND

With the Supreme Court's 1973 Roe v. Wade decision, which upheld the federal right to an abortion, abortion was first made lawful on a national level. In Whole Woman's Health v. Hellerstedt, the court ruled that states cannot enact abortion restrictions that place an "undue burden" on the procedure. The court then upheld that decision in 2017. However, the pro-abortion Guttmacher Institute reports that states have imposed more than 1,300 abortion restrictions since Roe v. Wade was decided in 1973, including more than 100 last year alone. Republican state lawmakers have repeatedly targeted abortion to persuade the Supreme Court to reconsider its precedent. As the conservative-leaning Supreme Court decided to take up the case against Mississippi's abortion ban and reevaluate Roe v. Wade in 2021, pro-lifers won several triumphs. When Texas' Senate Bill 8 (SB 8) went into effect on September 1 and effectively outlawed nearly all abortions after six weeks, the country's abortion laws became the strictest since Roe v. Wade. Idaho and Oklahoma have since adopted similar legislation.

Chapter 1

In the landmark decision Roe v. Wade, 410 U.S. 113 (1973), the U.S. Supreme Court determined that a pregnant woman's right to an abortion is generally protected by the U.S. Constitution. The ruling, which invalidated several federal and state abortion regulations in the US, sparked a national discussion about whether or how much abortion should be legal, who should make that decision and the proper place of morality and religion in politics. It also influenced discussions on the procedures the Supreme Court ought to follow when making constitutional rulings.

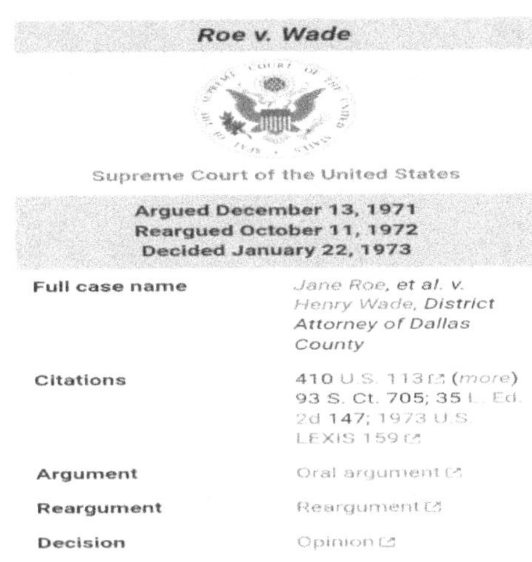

Case opinions	
Majority	Blackmun, joined by Burger, Douglas, Brennan, Stewart, Marshall, Powell
Concurrence	Burger
Concurrence	Douglas
Concurrence	Stewart
Dissent	White, joined by Rehnquist
Dissent	Rehnquist

Laws applied
U.S. Const. Amend. XIV; Tex. Code Crim. Proc. arts. 1191–94, 1196

Overruled by
Planned Parenthood v. Casey (1992) (in part), *Dobbs v. Jackson Women's Health Organization* (2022) (in full)

Norma McCorvey, who filed the lawsuit under the legal alias "Jane Roe," became expecting her third child in 1969. In Texas, where McCorvey resided, it was against the law to have an abortion unless it was essential to preserve the mother's life. Sarah Weddington and Linda Coffee, two of her attorneys, filed a lawsuit on her behalf in a federal court in the United States against Henry Wade, the district attorney in her community, claiming that Texas's abortion laws were unconstitutional. The relevant Texas abortion laws were deemed unconstitutional by a three-judge panel of the U.S. District Court for the Northern District of Texas in their favour. The United States Supreme Court heard an appeal from the parties over this decision.

The Due Process Clause of the Fourteenth Amendment to the United States Constitution establishes a basic "right to privacy," which safeguards a pregnant woman's right to an abortion, according to a 7-2 decision by the Supreme Court on January 22, 1973. The Court did, however, ruled that the right to an abortion is not unqualified and must be weighed against the interests of the state in safeguarding the health of women and unborn children. By setting a trimester timeline that will control all abortion laws in the US, the Court was able to reconcile these conflicting interests. Governments were only able to mandate that abortions be carried out by licensed medical professionals during the first trimester.

Governments may impose restrictions on abortions during the second trimester, but only to safeguard the health of the mother and not the fetus. Abortions might be controlled and even outlawed beyond viability (the third trimester and the final weeks of the second trimester), but only if the legislation made an exemption for abortions required to save the mother's "life" or "health." The Court further categorized the right to an abortion as "fundamental," which required courts to assess contested abortion restrictions using the strictest possible judicial review standards in the United States.

One of the most divisive rulings in American history was the Roe decision by the Supreme Court. For decades, pro-life politicians and activists fought to overturn the judgment. Although Planned Parenthood v. Casey overturned Roe's trimester framework and dropped Roe's "strict scrutiny" requirement in favour of a more flexible "undue burden" test, the Supreme Court upheld its "central holding" in that case notwithstanding criticism of Roe.

The Dobbs v. Jackson final ruling, released on June 24, 2022, said that "the Constitution does not provide a right to abortion" and that "the ability to restrict abortion is restored to the people and their elected representatives." Casey and Roe were both overturned.

Chapter 2

How Americans Feel About Abortion in Roe v. Wade

While a review of national polls reveals many Americans consistently split between identifying with the partisan labels "pro-choice" or "pro-life," a clear majority supports keeping the procedure legal—though that support drops quickly depending on the circumstance. The Supreme Court overturned Roe v. Wade, allowing states to outlaw abortion.

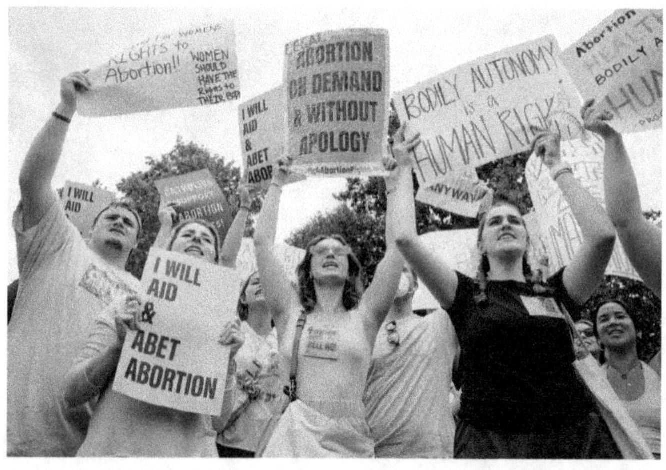

Widespread support for abortion rights: Gallup polls show that Americans support abortion in all or most circumstances at 80 per cent in May 2021, only marginally higher than in 1975 (76 per cent), and the Pew Research Center finds that 59 per cent of adults believe abortion should be legal, down from 60 per cent in 1995—though there has been fluctuation, with support falling to a low of 47 per cent in 2009.

A Quinnipiac poll indicated support for abortion being legal in all or most situations hit a near-record high in September with 63per cent support, while the percentage of Americans who feel abortion is morally acceptable rose to a record high of 47 per cent in May from a record low of 36 per cent in 2009.

Consistent support for Roe: A November Quinnipiac survey found that 63 per cent of respondents agreed with the court's decision; a January Marquette Law School poll found that 72 percent of respondents did, and a January CNN poll found that 69 per cent of respondents disagreed.

If Roe is overturned, according to a January CNN survey, 59 per cent of respondents want their state's abortion regulations to be "more permissive than restrictive," while only 20 per cent want an outright ban (another 20 per cent want it to be restricted but not banned).

Strongest pro-abortion sentiment—within reason: According to a June poll by the Associated Press/NORC, 87% of respondents support abortion when the woman's life is in jeopardy, 84% support exceptions for rape or incest, and 74% support abortion if the child is would be born with a fatal condition.

When abortion support declines: As the pregnancy progresses. According to AP/NORC, 61 per cent of people believe abortion should be legal in the first trimester, but only 34 per cent and 19 per cent do so in the second and third. A Wall Street Journal poll conducted in April also revealed that more people support banning abortions at 15 weeks of pregnancy than oppose it.

Partisan split, but not always: Democrats are statistically much more likely to support abortion rights than Republicans, with Quinnipiac finding in September that only 39% of Republicans believe abortion should be legal in all or most cases, compared to 189% of Democrats. However, exceptions for rape and incest and when the mother's life is in danger are supported by 70% and 76% of Republicans, respectively.

A higher percentage of every religious group surveyed, including white non-evangelicals, Black Protestants, and Catholics, support abortion rights, except white evangelical Protestants (77 per cent of whom believe abortion should be illegal). Pew found that Americans with religious affiliations are much more likely to oppose abortion than the nonreligious (82 per cent of whom believe abortion should be legal).

Not as significant a gender divide as you may imagine Pew found that 62 per cent of women want abortion to be legal, compared to 56 per cent of men, suggesting that women are slightly more inclined than men to support abortion.

Asian Americans are the most supportive: According to Pew's poll, most people of all races believe that abortion should be legal. However, support was higher among Black respondents (who believe it should be legal) and Asian respondents (who believe it should be legal) than it was among White and Hispanic respondents (57 per cent and 58 per cent respectively).

Age affects support: According to the Pew research, support for abortion is strongest among those between the ages of 18 and 29 (67 per cent feel it should be legal), compared to 61 per cent for those between 30 and 49, 53 per cent for those between 50 and 64, and 55 per cent for those 65 and over.

A Washington Post/ABC poll found a similar correlation: support rises with higher levels of education, with 68 per cent of college graduates favouring legalization compared to 61 per cent of those with some college and 50 per cent with only a high school diploma or less.

Parents are less likely to support abortion rights: A September poll by All In Together, Lake Research, and Emerson College Polling found that 58 per cent of parents want the Supreme Court to uphold Roe v. Wade, compared to 62 per cent of non-parents, while only 36 per cent of those with children in the home opposed the Texas near-total abortion ban.

Cities are more likely to support Roe v. Wade (with a support rate of 69 per cent) than residents of suburban or rural areas. The Northeast is the region with the highest support for abortion rights, with 71 per cent of residents wanting Roe v. Wade to be upheld, compared to 58 per cent in the Midwest, 53 per cent in the South, and 66 per cent in the West (56 per cent and 57ppeccentpectively).

Support increases with income level: According to a Post/ABC poll, 59 per cent of respondents who make less than $50,000 annually want the court to uphold the legislation, compared to 62 per cent of respondents who make between $50,000 and $100,000 and 65 percent of respondents who make more than $100,000.

Chapter 3

Reactions of women who support abortion rights according to the New York Times

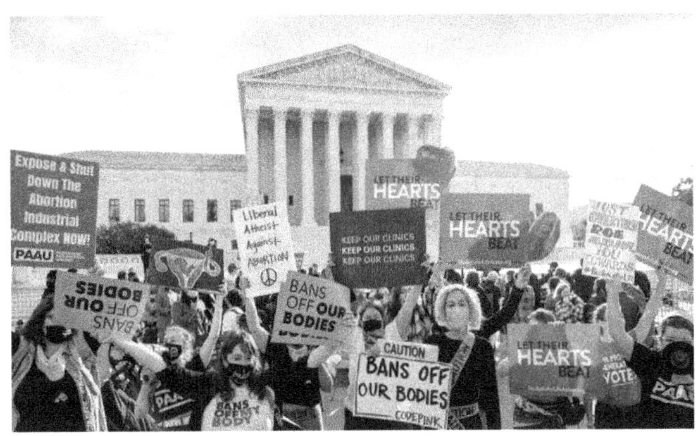

As they respond to Friday's Supreme Court ruling overturning Roe v. Wade, our correspondents are chatting with women all around the country. Here is a sample of what they have learned from female proponents of preserving access to abortion.

Thinking of the next generation of young women

One of the first things Nicole Stipp, 37, did after hearing the decision was text her younger sister and her sister-in-law, both in their 20s. Nicole is a co-owner of Trouble Bar in Louisville and a volunteer for the Kentucky Health Justice Network's abortion hotline.

Ms Stipp, who herself has had abortions, said, "They're very vulnerable." It's absurd to believe that as of this morning, my younger sister has fewer rights than I have. Abortion has always been available to me. Legislation hasn't made it simple or unhindered, but the fact that my 25-year-old sister no longer has that right is unsettling.

'Women should have the choice'

Litzy Morales, who was accompanying her 2-year-old daughter in a stroller to Grand Park in downtown Los Angeles, said, "Every child deserves to have a happy household." "I feel for all the mothers who are forced to bear children they are unable to care for and who are unsure of what will happen next," she said.

As a former victim of sexual assault, Ms Morales expressed concern that the Supreme Court's decision would be particularly challenging for rape victims.

For women to not be able to control how their lives turn out if something uncontrollable and unintended happens to them is "extremely painful to go through," Ms Morales said. "Women should have the freedom to choose whether or not they are prepared to care for a child."

A fear that a lack of access to abortion will lead to deaths

Denise Taylor, a community health centre employee with 11 locations in the predominantly rural Mississippi Delta, said on Friday that she was devastated by the Supreme Court's decision and was holding back tears.

Many women would die as a result of illegal abortions, according to Ms Taylor. "A woman's body is her own, and the court has no jurisdiction to instruct her what to do with it."

'The decision has set women back at least 100 years

The decision "outraged," according to Jennifer White, 41, of Sioux Falls, South Dakota, and she believes others should feel the same way.

According to Ms White, "I think the decision has set women back at least 100 years." South Dakotan women, at least.

Ms White, a painter, gallery owner, and member of the Arikara tribe claimed that South Dakota's female government officials, including Republican Governor Kristi Noem, had let her down.

"I'm putting a lot of pressure on it because I'm frustrated that women don't see the needs of other women," she said. "We struggled for a voice for a very long time, especially women of colour like me. Furthermore, it is absurd to watch our power being transferred.

A Mississippi woman reacts with anger, but not disbelief

"I knew this was coming but I didn't expect to feel such anger," said Amalie Hahn, 49, of Jackson, Miss. "The very first emotion I had was anger. I could say I don't believe this is happening, but I do believe this is happening. I do believe this is the American way. I don't think we women have ever mattered. I have been trying to figure out a way to process my anger, process my fear."

"You want to ban abortions in the state of Mississippi, but you don't want to take into account that Mississippi is one of, if not the worst, state to give birth in," Ms Hahn added. "We are amid a formula shortage and poverty is at an all-time high and they are forcing women to have babies. This is insane."

'The nation is on fire'

Hannah Drake, 45, a poet and writer in Louisville, Ky., heard the news of the Roe ruling as she was about to attend a virtual meeting.

"The nation is on fire, so this meeting is not relevant right now," MsDrake said she thought at the time. "A rock just landed in the ocean and the ripple this will have — anything else today is insignificant because this doesn't just stop at one thing. Next, let's look at Brown v. The Board of Education, and s age. It will not end with this."

Ms Drake said that she expected that Black women like herself would be the ones who faced the most severe ramifications of the decision. "Now we have to deal with this thing and we don't have the resources," she said. "We will not have excellent health care, an underground doctor, a private hospital, or the friend of a friend who can help you out."

Ms Drake said she chose to have a daughter at 19 and attempted to have an abortion in her late 30s, but when she arrived at a clinic her car was swarmed by protesters. Overwhelmed, she started crying, left the parking lot, and drove home, she said. A week later she had a miscarriage, alone, without medical support, in a bathroom stall at work.

Chapter 4

SURPRISING FACT

The percentage of Americans who identify as "pro-choice" or "pro-life" has not changed since 1995, despite support for whether abortion should be legal remaining largely consistent over that time. In comparison to the 56 per cent and 33 per cent who stated the same in 1995, respectively, Gallup reported that 49 per cent and 47 per cent of Americans today identify as pro-choice and pro-life, respectively. Although the majority of Americans have at least occasionally backed the legalization of abortion, in 2019, 2013, 2012, 2010 and 2009, more respondents identified as pro-life than pro-choice.

According to a May 2021 Ipsos poll, 66 per cent of Americans believe abortion should be legal in some situations, compared to a global average of 71 per cent. This indicates that Americans' support for abortion lags far behind that of many other nations. The countries with abortion views that rank lower than the United States are Brazil, India, South Africa, Colombia, Mexico, Turkey, Peru, and Malaysia. Support for abortion is highest in Sweden (88 per cent support), the Netherlands (85 per cent support), and France (81 per cent support).

Where Abortion Legislation Stands Across the U.S.

Several states have imposed restrictions on abortion, while others have reinforced their ability to provide the procedure. Here is a look at some recent developments:

Restricting Abortion

Oklahoma: Gov. Kevin Stitt signed a bill that bans nearly all abortions starting at fertilization. The new law, which takes effect immediately, is the most restrictive abortion ban in the country.

Florida: In March, Gov. Ron DeSantis signed into law a ban on most abortions after 15 weeks of pregnancy. It takes effect on July 1.

Idaho: A ban on abortion after six weeks of pregnancy was set to take effect on April 22 but has been temporarily blocked by the Idaho Supreme Court.

Kentucky: Lawmakers overrode the governor's veto of a law restricting abortion after 15 weeks. A federal judge temporarily blocked the measure.

Reinforcing Abortion

California: Abortion rights are already protected in the State Constitution, but lawmakers proposed an amendment to bolster those protections. A package of bills also seeks to make the state a "refuge" for women seeking abortions.

Connecticut: A new law would shield abortion providers and patients from lawsuits initiated by states that have banned or plan to ban abortion.

New York: Several bills have been introduced to strengthen abortion rights, including one that would create an abortion access fund.

Maryland: Overriding the governor's veto, lawmakers passed a bill that allows trained medical professionals other than physicians to perform abortions.

State laws regarding Roe

There have been numerous abortion-related laws at the state level. Most states passed legislation safeguarding healthcare professionals with a conscientious objection to abortion in the decade after Roe. Before Roe v. Wade, nine states had previously passed laws granting statutory protection to people who did not want to conduct or participate in abortions. As of 2011, there was legislation in 47 states plus the District of Columbia that permitted some people to refuse to carry out specific tasks or share information regarding abortion or reproductive health.

The Church Amendment of 1973 was put up at the federal level to shield private hospitals that opposed abortion from losing funding. It first passed the Senate by a vote of 92-1, then the House by a vote of 372-1, and finally the Senate by a vote of 94-0 for the final bill that contained it. Justice Blackmun backed this law as well as others safeguarding certain doctors and entire hospitals run by religious organizations.

If Roe v. Wade is repealed, some states have passed legislation to keep abortion lawful. California, Connecticut, Hawaii, Maine, Maryland, Nevada, and Washington are among those states. Other states have passed "trigger laws" that would go into effect if Roe v. Wade were to be reversed and have the effect of prohibiting abortions on a state-by-state basis. These states are North Dakota, South Dakota, Kentucky, Louisiana, Mississippi, and

Arkansas. Furthermore, several states did not repeal anti-abortion laws before 1973, and some of those laws might be reinstated if Roe were overturned.

Mississippi House Bill 1390 was ratified on April 16, 2012. Without having to invalidate Roe v. Wade, the bill tried to make abortion impossible. On July 13, 2012, in the United States District Court for the Southern District of Mississippi Judge Daniel Porter Jordan III issued an injunction against the law. On April 15, 2013, he granted a new injunction that only related to the portion of the law requiring hospital admitting privileges for the person performing the abortions. Despite Judge Emilio M. Garza's dissent, a three-judge panel from the U.S. Court of Appeals for the Fifth Circuit upheld the injunction against a portion of the law on July 29, 2014. The decision, which was made "almost fifty years before the right to an abortion was discovered in the penumbra of the Constitution," specifically cited a case unconnected to Roe. Mississippi petitioned the Supreme Court to consider the case on February 18, 2015, but on June 28, 2016, they decided not to.

On May 14, 2019, Alabama Governor Kay Ivey signed the Human Life Protection Act to repeal Roe v. Wade to the Supreme Court. If it becomes law, it will make abortion a crime for the abortion doctor, with the exclusions of major health risks to the mother or fatal fetal anomalies. Abortion recipients will not be held legally accountable in either a criminal or civil capacity. A preliminary injunction against the law was issued by Judge Myron Thompson of the U.S. District Court for the Northern District of Alabama on October 29, 2019.

The Texas Heartbeat Act, passed by Texas Legislature in May 2021, outlaws abortions except in life-threatening situations as soon as a fetal heartbeat is discovered. This generally occurs as early as six weeks into pregnancy, frequently before women are even aware that they are expecting. The statute established that anybody residing in Texas who is not an employee or official of a state or municipal government may file a lawsuit against abortion facilities and medical professionals who are "aiding and abetting" abortion procedures after six weeks. A provision prohibits legal action against someone who caused an abortion patient to get pregnant by rape, sexual assault, or incest. The law was enacted on September 1, 2021, and the U.S. Supreme Court rejected a request to stop its enforcement on that day in a 5-4 decision. The Court once more refused to stop the law's implementation on October 22, 2021 and decided to hear the arguments in the United States v. Texas (2021) on November 1 of that same year. They restricted the inquiry to a standing review. The lawsuit was dismissed by the court on December 10, 2021, because it should not have been accepted by lower courts. This ruling permits legal action against the executive commissioner of the Texas Health and Human Services Commission as well as the executive directors of the state's licensing boards for medicine, nursing, and pharmacy, but bars certain other legal actions that aim to invalidate the legislation.